Cannabis Use
and Mental Health

Cannabis Use and Mental Health

A Critical Review of Risks and Benefits

North Carolina Psychiatric Association

Content editing by Thomas Penders, MD, MS, DLFAPA

Library of Congress Control Number: 2016920805
ISBN: Hardcover   978-1-5245-6971-6
               Softcover   978-1-5245-6970-9
               eBook   978-1-5245-6969-3

Print information available on the last page.

Rev. date: 03/09/2017

To order additional copies of this book, contact:
Xlibris
1-888-795-4274
www.Xlibris.com
Orders@Xlibris.com
732599

CONTENTS

Introduction

Several recent public opinion polls support the observation that attitudes toward the legalization of botanical cannabis products have changed dramatically over the past decade.[1] At the start of 2017 the citizens of 28 states, the District of Columbia and Guam may use some form of marijuana legally. Eight states have passed legislation regulating recreational sale and use of Cannabis. As the first state to legalize marijuana, Colorado has witnessed the sale of over $1 billion of marijuana products in the most recent year. The state of Colorado collected $135 million in tax revenue from these sales. Since public attitudes toward liberalization are more pervasive among younger voters, it seems inevitable that the momentum for further relaxation of restrictions on marijuana will continue. Concurrently, prevalence of use of marijuana has doubled over the decade from 2002 to 2013.[2]

Public policy decisions relating to this phenomenon are complex and include implications for all institutions of society from law enforcement to public health and health care delivery. Constructive public debate about the pros and cons of liberalization must be informed by an understanding of what science has learned about the risks and benefits to health in different population groups. On September 21, 2015, the American Society of Addiction Medicine (ASAM) issued a new policy statement on marijuana, cannabinoids, and legalization that favors a more balanced response to legalization efforts.

This monograph, conceived and written by psychiatrist members of the North Carolina Psychiatric Association and supported by the Psychiatric Foundation of North Carolina, is intended to meet the need for a summary statement of what is known from scientific research efforts about the effects of use of cannabis products on the mental health of those who are using at varying ages and levels of vulnerability.

Notes

1. Pew Research Center. In debate over legalizing marijuana, disagreement over drug's dangers. http://www.people-press.org/2015/04/14/in-debate-over-legalizing-marijuana-disagreement-over-drugs-dangers/.

2. Hasin, D., Saha, T. D., Kerridge, B. T., et al. Prevalence of marijuana use disorders in the United States between 2001–2012 and 2012–2013, *JAMA Psychiatry*. 2015;72(12):1235–42.

About the North Carolina Psychiatric Association

The North Carolina Psychiatric Association (NCPA) is a professional medical organization that represents more than 900 psychiatrists statewide; it is the district branch of the American Psychiatric Association. NCPA's mission is to promote the highest-quality care for North Carolina residents with mental illness, including substance use disorders; advance and represent the profession of psychiatry and medicine in North Carolina; and serve the professional needs of its membership.

About the Psychiatric Foundation of North Carolina

The Psychiatric Foundation of North Carolina is a 501(c)3 organization, and its primary goals focus on providing training, education, and research that assists psychiatrists in offering the best possible care for patients. It also works to educate the public about psychiatry; psychiatric illnesses, including their signs and symptoms; and treatments.

About the Authors

Ureh Nena Lekwauwa, MD, DFAPA, is the recent medical director, North Carolina's Department of Health and Human Services, Division of Mental Health, Developmental Disabilities, and Substance Abuse Services.

Chelsea L. Neumann, MD, is currently a PGY-5, first-year fellow at the Warren Alpert Medical School at Brown University Child and Adolescent Psychiatry Training Program. During her last two years of psychiatry residency at Duke University, she worked in Durham, North Carolina, at Triangle Residential Options for Substance Abusers providing psychiatric treatment to individuals with substance use disorders, during which time she collaborated with Dr. Ashwin

Patkar to complete a review of the current literature outlining the effects of cannabis on physical and mental health. She has continued research interests in the effects of cannabis use on medical and psychiatric conditions and is currently researching the correlation between the quantity of cannabis use and depressed mood in adolescents.

Heather N. Oxentine, MD, is a recent graduate of the psychiatric residency program at East Carolina University's Brody School of Medicine. She is currently a Fellow in Addiction Psychiatry at Emory University. Her clinical experience includes research related to cannabis use either as a primary or as a secondary diagnosis. Further, Dr. Oxentine is interested in continuing research related to political and medical implications regarding the legalization of cannabis.

Ashwin A. Patkar, MD, DFAPA, MRCPsych, DFASAM, is professor of psychiatry and community and family medicine at Duke University Medical Center in Durham, North Carolina. Dr. Patkar is the medical director of Duke Addictions Program and Duke Center of Addictive Behavior. He has over 20 years of clinical and research experience in addictions.

Thomas Penders, MD, MS, DLFAPA, is an affiliate associate professor of psychiatry at the Brody School of Medicine at East Carolina University. He is the president of the North Carolina Psychiatric Association and the past Addictions Committee chair.

Diana O. Perkins, MD, MPH, DFAPA, is professor of psychiatry at the University of North Carolina at Chapel Hill. One of the founders and is the medical director of Outreach and Support Intervention Services (OASIS), one of the first Coordinated Specialty Care programs serving persons in the early stages of a psychotic disorder or at high risk for a psychotic disorder. The mission of OASIS is to foster sustained recovery and prevent disability from psychosis. Her research interests focus on discovering factors that contribute to psychosis vulnerability and finding better treatments for psychotic disorders.

P.G. Shelton, MD, FAPA, is an assistant professor of child and adolescent psychiatry at East Carolina University's Brody School of Medicine.

Marijuana Use Trends and Psychiatric Disorders

Thomas Penders, MD, MS, DLFAPA

History

The hemp plant *Cannabis sativa* is among the oldest known to humankind. Evidence for its use as a source of fiber for clothing and rope and in the production of parchments can be traced to Central Asia 12,000 years ago. The word "canvas" is derived from cannabis. Throughout human history, extracts of the cannabis plant have been used as medicine for a variety of conditions, such as muscle spasm, nausea, and nervous disorders. Its introduction into Western medicine is attributed to an English army surgeon, William O'Shaughnessy, who used cannabis extracts while in India during his appointment as physician and director of telegraphy with the East India Company in 1844. Cannabis plants accompanied the settlers who arrived at Jamestown in 1607. During colonial times, and continuing for the next 300 years, extracts of the cannabis plant had been used by physicians and the public for treatment of a variety of musculoskeletal, digestive, and nervous conditions. Various nostrums, including extracts of cannabis, were freely available to the public unregulated and widely used in popular cures.[1]

The first effort to control the sale of cannabis products, the Marijuana Tax Act, became federal law in 1937 over the objections of the American Medical Association. Over the remainder of the century, increasing regulation by federal and state governments culminated in inclusion of cannabis as a schedule I drug with high abuse potential and no accepted medical use by the Controlled Substances Act of 1970. Despite this, very limited numbers of individuals have received medical marijuana as part of a tightly controlled compassionate use program administered by the National Institute of Drug Abuse.

Recent Use Trends

Each year researchers from the Department of Social Sciences at the University of Michigan survey about 50,000 secondary students about their use of alcohol and illicit drugs. In 2012, about half (49 percent) of high school seniors reported the use of an illicit drug. For 10th and 8th graders, the figures were 37 percent and 15 percent, respectively. In the vast majority of cases, the drug reported was marijuana. Strikingly, about 1 in 15 12th graders indicated that they used marijuana on a daily basis last year. Among adults in America, despite a leveling off of the prevalence of illicit drug use in general, about 7 percent of the US population use marijuana at least monthly, a figure that has grown each year out of the past five. Among high school–age children, marijuana use in the past month exceeds use of tobacco products.[2]

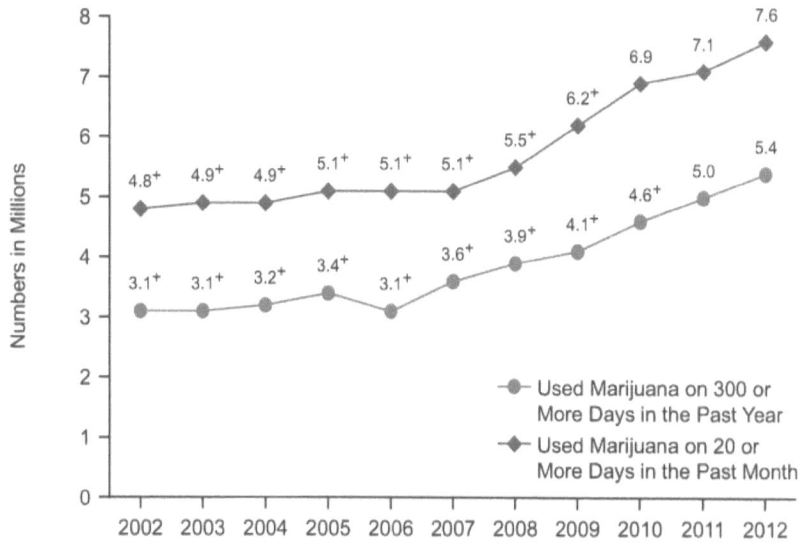

After alcohol and tobacco, marijuana is regularly reported to have the highest rates of dependence and abuse in national surveys. In 2011, 4.2 million individuals qualified under DSM-IV TR for a diagnosis of cannabis abuse or dependence. Individuals with diagnosed mental disorders use marijuana at rates that are seven times more than those who do not have a mental disorder.[3] Among patients in treatment for psychiatric disorders, there is a tenfold increase in marijuana use disorders as compared with the general population. These statistics underline the important observation that patients in psychiatric treatment are more likely to use, tend to use more, and are more likely to become dependent on this widely available substance.[4]

Public Attitudes and Legislative Changes

Public attitudes and views of the dangerousness of cannabis are changing. These attitudes have had an important effect on public policies and legislations related to the use of marijuana. Over the past decade, about half of our states have either decriminalized or greatly reduced the penalties for possession and use of small amounts of cannabis products. Four states have passed legislations providing for legalization for recreational purposes, and in 23 states where it has been made available for "medical purposes," use appears to be rapidly expanding fueled by robust cottage industries in provision of numbers of products that include cannabis.[5] Today there are a few counties that derive the majority of their tax revenue from sales of legal cannabis.

Paradoxically, arrests for possession and sale of marijuana have trended upward recently.[6] An average of 100 individuals are detained per hour nationally as reported by FBI statistics. This is occurring despite the announcement by the US Department of Justice that they would not prosecute those using cannabis within the legal structure of the laws of those states. Canada has recently approved an expansion in a regulated system of marijuana culture that has an estimated revenue potential of $1.3 billion according to executives of Tweed, a corporate producer of medical marijuana. It is estimated that over the next decade, there will be 500,000 users of the product among our northern neighbors.

Legal Status in North Carolina

Here in North Carolina where use of small amounts of marijuana remains a class 3 misdemeanor, a bill to downgrade this to a summary offense was defeated in the past legislative session.[7] The American Civil Liberties Union has recently reported a dramatic disparity in the prosecution of users of marijuana. In North Carolina, 50 percent of those prosecuted have been African American. The future of the legal status of this curious plant is now under intense scrutiny. Opinions on public policy range from support for full legalization to continue restriction and control.

In North Carolina, House Bill 84 (Enact Medical Cannabis Act) received a rare negative report and was dead for the 2013–2014 session. News reports indicated that legislators were being "harassed" by constituents almost all of whom were in favor of passage. Groups advocating availability of medical marijuana have been formed and are growing in our state. The listing of marijuana as a schedule I drug under the Controlled Substances Act defining it as a substance with no currently accepted medical use and a high potential for abuse is a source of increasing controversy.

The Epilepsy Alternative Treatment Act, effective in 2014, supports research under the oversight of the Department of Health and Human Services.

Cannabis as Medications

Since the discovery that tetrahydrocannabinol (THC) is the active ingredient in smoked marijuana, there has been research interest at both clinical and basic science levels in the use of cannabis as a potential therapeutic agent. Discovery and elaboration of the endogenous endocannabinoid system and its role in modulating stress in health and disease promises to provide insights into therapeutic applications for a variety of problems, such as treatment of pain, obesity, muscle spasms, and seizures. Additionally, growing information is pointing to deleterious effects of cannabinoids. Multiple studies have now demonstrated increased risk for development of schizophrenic-like psychosis among youth who are regular users of smoked cannabis.

The accumulated body of evidence relating to the positive and negative health effects of marijuana has great relevance for the current debate about liberalizing availability of cannabis products. The North Carolina Psychiatric Association Addictions Committee will present clinical information for our members.

Notes

1. Bostwick, J. M. Blurred boundaries: The therapeutics and politics of medical marijuana. *Proceedings of Mayo Clinic.* 2012;87(2):172–186.

2. Johnston, L. D., O'Malley, P. M., Miech, R. A., Bachman, J. G., and Schulenberg, J. E. *Monitoring the future national survey results on drug use, 1975–2015: Overview, key findings on adolescent drug use.* Ann Arbor: Institute for Social Research, University of Michigan, 2016.

3. Wittchen, H. U., Frohlich, C., Behrendt, S., et al. Cannabis use and cannabis use disorders and their relationship to mental disorders: A ten-year prospective-longitudinal community study in adolescents. *Drug and Alcohol Dependence.* April 2007;88 Suppl 1:S60–70.

4. Semple, D. M., McIntosh, A. M., and Lawrie, S. M. Cannabis as a risk factor for psychosis: A systematic review. *Journal of Psychopharmacology.* 2005;19(2):187–94.

5. Hasin, D. S., Saha, T. D., Kerridge, B. T., et al. Prevalence of marijuana use disorders in the United States between 2001–2002 and 2012–2013. *JAMA Psychiatry.* 2015;72(12):123–1242.

6. Chu, Y. W. The effects of medical marijuana use on illegal marijuana use. *Journal of Health Economics.* 2014;38:43–61.

7. National Conference of State Legislators. State Medical Marijuana Laws. Retrieved February 20, 2016, from http://www.ncsl.org/research/health/state-medical-marijuana-laws.aspx

Marijuana and Psychosis

Diana O. Perkins, MD, MPH, DFAPA

Marijuana use, especially a pattern of use that begins during early adolescence, or heavy use in late adolescence or early adulthood, has emerged as an environmental risk factor for the development of psychosis, increasing risk about fourfold.[1,2,3,4,5] This means that about 4 percent of heavy or early marijuana users will develop schizophrenia, compared with about 1 percent of the general population. Thus, marijuana may increase the risk of schizophrenia, but only in persons who have a biological vulnerability. These studies also suggest that, given current rates of marijuana use, marijuana likely plays a causal role in about 10–14 percent of all cases of schizophrenia.[6]

Interestingly, at the first episode of psychosis, the "kind" of schizophrenia associated with marijuana use is characterized by less severe negative symptoms and cognitive impairments[7,8] as well as an earlier age of onset.[9] It is currently unclear if these differences in presentation are due to marijuana exerting some therapeutic benefit, that the type of schizophrenia where marijuana is a risk factor is a more benign disorder than the type of schizophrenia that develops for other reasons, that obtaining marijuana use requires intact social skills, or some other confounding factor. However, once schizophrenia develops, continued use of marijuana is associated with relapse, rehospitalization, and worse functional outcomes.[10,11] For this reason, substance abuse treatment is a critical component of the care of persons with schizophrenia who use marijuana.

The brain's own cannabinoid system, termed the endocannabinoid system, is a key regulator of neurotransmitter release (including dopamine, GABA, and glutamate) and neuronal plasticity.[12] The endocannabinoid system is now known to regulate recovery of the endocrine and autonomic nervous system from stress, immune system function, and energy balance. The endocannabinoid system also plays key roles in neurodevelopment. Marijuana contains multiple cannabinoids, with the main cannabinoid delta-9-tetrahydrahydrocannabinol (THC). THC is a "partial agonist" at cannabinoid receptors in the brain and thus activates these receptors. THC is a prime suspect to explain the effect of marijuana on psychosis, based on evidence that THC administration induces a transient psychosis in healthy persons as well as persons with schizophrenia.[13] This idea has led to trials of cannabinoid receptor antagonists, such as rimonabant, in schizophrenia, that unfortunately have failed thus far to show clinical benefits.[14]

Cannabis also contains cannabidiol (CBD), which is reported to have antianxiety and antipsychotic effects and to protect against the psychosis-inducing effects of THC.[15] CBD appears to have very weak effects on cannabinoid receptors but has been shown to influence the metabolism of the body's own cannabinoid, anandamide, increasing anandamide levels. A recent 4-week double-blind clinical trial in 42 patients with acute psychosis compared CBD to amisulpride (an antipsychotic available in Europe).[16] In this study, CBD was comparable with amisulpride in reduction of total, positive, and negative symptoms and was not associated with extrapyramidal side effects, weight gain, or prolactin elevation. CBD treatment was also associated with elevations in blood levels of anandamide, and change in anandamide levels was highly and significantly correlated with symptom change. The authors advance the intriguing theory that anandamide is protective against psychosis and that the CBD mechanism of action is to interfere with anandamide metabolism and thus boost anandamide levels.

In summary, marijuana contains a complex mixture of potential active compounds, with THC and CBD seeming to have opposing effects relative to psychosis. Use of marijuana in childhood or adolescence or heavy use in young adulthood appears to increase risk of schizophrenia by about fourfold, with THC the likely culprit. The effect of increasing use of marijuana in adolescents together with the increasing concentrations of THC relative to CBD in strains of marijuana raise concerns that the relative contribution of marijuana to development of schizophrenia could increase in the future. The endocannabinoid system is emerging as an intriguing treatment target in persons with schizophrenia, with CBD in particular showing early promise as an effective drug.

Notes

1. Manrique-Garcia, E., Zammit, S., Dalman, C., Hemmingsson, T., Andreasson, S., and Allebeck, P. Cannabis, schizophrenia and other non-affective psychoses: 35 years of follow-up of a population-based cohort. *Psychological Medicine.* 2012;42(6):1321–8.

2. Davis, G. P., Compton, M. T., Wang, S., Levin, F. R., and Blanco, C. Association between cannabis use, psychosis, and schizotypal personality disorder: Findings from the National Epidemiologic Survey on Alcohol and Related Conditions. *Schizophrenia Research.* 2013;151(1–3):197–202.

3. Hickman, M., Vickerman, P., Macleod, J., Kirkbride, J., and Jones, P. B. Cannabis and schizophrenia: Model

projections of the impact of the rise in cannabis use on historical and future trends in schizophrenia in England and Wales. *Addiction* (Abingdon, England). 2007;102(4):597–606.

4. Arseneault, L., Cannon, M., Poulton, R., Murray, R., Caspi, A., and Moffitt, T. E. Cannabis use in adolescence and risk for adult psychosis: Longitudinal prospective study. *BMJ* (Clinical research ed.). 2002;325(7374):1212–3.

5. Van Os, J., Bak, M., Hanssen, M., Bijl, R. V., de Graaf, R., and Verdoux, H. Cannabis use and psychosis: A longitudinal population-based study. *American Journal of Epidemiology*. 2002;156(4):319–27.

6. Moore, T. H., Zammit, S., Lingford-Hughes, A., Barnes, T. R., Jones, P. B., Burke, M., et al. Cannabis use and risk of psychotic or affective mental health outcomes: A systematic review. *Lancet*. 2007;370(9584):319–28.

7. Segev, A., and Lev-Ran, S. Neurocognitive functioning and cannabis use in schizophrenia. *Curr Pharm Des.* 2012;18(32):4999–5007.

8. Burns, J. K., Jhazbhay, K., and Emsley, R. Cannabis use predicts shorter duration of untreated psychosis and lower levels of negative symptoms in first-episode psychosis: A South African study. *African Journal of Psychiatry.* 2010;13(5):395–9.

9. Donoghue, K., Doody, G. A., Murray, R. M., Jones, P. B., Morgan, C., Dazzan, P., et al. Cannabis use, gender, and age of onset of schizophrenia: Data from the AESOP study. *Psychiatry Research.* 2014.

10. D'Souza, D. C., Sewell, R. A., and Ranganathan, M. Cannabis and psychosis/schizophrenia: Human studies. *European Archives of Psychiatry and Clinical Neuroscience.* 2009;259(7):413–31.

11. Faber, G., Smid, H. G., Van Gool, A. R., Wunderink, L., van den Bosch, R. J., and Wiersma, D. Continued cannabis use and outcome in first-episode psychosis:

Data from a randomized, open-label, controlled trial. *The Journal of Clinical Psychiatry.* 2012;73(5):632–8.

12.   Castillo, P. E., Younts, T. J., Chavez, A. E., and Hashimotodani, Y. Endocannabinoid signaling and synaptic function. *Neuron.* 2012;76(1):70–81.

13.   D'Souza, D. C., Sewell, R. A., and Ranganathan, M. Cannabis and psychosis/schizophrenia: Human studies. *European Archives of Psychiatry and Clinical Neuroscience.* 2009;259(7):413–31.

14.   Roser, P., and Haussleiter, I. S. Antipsychotic-like effects of cannabidiol and rimonabant: Systematic review of animal and human studies. *Curr Pharm Des.* 2012;18(32):5141–55.

15.   Schubart, C. D., Sommer, I. E., Fusar-Poli, P., de Witte, L., Kahn, R. S., and Boks, M. P. Cannabidiol as a potential treatment for psychosis. *Eur Neuropsychopharmacol.* 2014;24(1):51–64.

16.   Leweke, F. M., Piomelli, D., Pahlisch, F., Muhl, D., Gerth, C. W., Hoyer, C., et al. Cannabidiol enhances anandamide signaling and alleviates psychotic symptoms of schizophrenia. *Transl Psychiatry.* 2012;2:e94.

Cannabis: Pharmacology, Psychoactive Agents, and Drug Interactions

Ureh Nena Lekwauwa, MD, DFAPA

Introduction

Cannabis or marijuana is the most commonly used illegal substance in the world, and approximately 4 percent of the world's population has used cannabis at least once in the past year.[1] Herbal cannabis contains over 400 compounds, including 60-plus cannabinoids that are aryl-substituted meroterpenes from the plant genus *Cannabis*.[2] Cannabidiol (CBD) is one of the 60 active cannabinoids identified in cannabis.[3] As a major component of the plant, CBD accounts for up to 40 percent of the plant's extract, as a nonpsychotropic phytocannabinoid. Pharmacology for most of the cannabinoids is largely unknown, but the potent psychoactive agent, tetrahydrocannabinol (THC), is the major psychoactive agent that has been isolated, synthesized, and studied. The effects of THC are dose-related, and most research on cannabis was established in the 1970s using smaller doses of 5–25 mg THC; therefore, the risks and consequences of today's marijuana use may be unknown because sophisticated cultivation in the past 30 years increased the potency of cannabis products. In the 1960s and 1970s, the average "reefer" contained about 10 mg THC.[4] Now "joints" made of skunkweed, netherweed, and other potent subspecies of *Cannabis sativa* can contain up to 150 mg of THC (or 300 mg if laced with hashish oil). Today's cannabis smoker may be exposed to THC doses many times greater than in the past. For every cannabis user who develops a dependency, in DSM-5 terminology, a moderate to severe cannabis disorder, 10 users do not.[5]

Cannabis Pharmacology

Pharmacokinetics

When smoked, 50 percent of THC in a joint is inhaled, and nearly all is absorbed through the lungs, rapidly entering the bloodstream and reaching the brain in minutes. The effects are perceptible within seconds and fully within minutes. With oral ingestion, bioavailability is lessened, and blood concentrations reach 25–39 percent of that obtained by smoking the same amount because of slow oral absorption and first metabolism in the liver. Once absorbed, THC and other cannabinoids are rapidly distributed to all tissues at rates dependent on the blood flow.

Cannabinoids are extremely lipid soluble and accumulate in fatty tissues, reaching peak concentrations in four to five days, and then are released slowly back into other body compartments, including the brain. Because THC is sequestered in fat, THC tissue elimination half-life is about seven days, and the complete elimination of a single dose may take up to 30 days. With repeated doses, high levels of cannabis accumulate in the body. In the brain, THC and other cannabinoids are differentially distributed—with high concentrations found in the neocortical, limbic, sensory, and motor areas.[6]

Cannabinoids are metabolized in the liver, resulting in more than 20 metabolites—some are active and have long half-lives, the major one being 11-hydroxy-THC. Many metabolites are excreted in urine, and some are excreted into the gut where they are reabsorbed and prolong cannabis actions. As a result of this delay and sequestering in fat, there is a poor relationship between plasma or urine concentrations and degree of cannabinoid-induced intoxication. The 11-hydroxy-THC is rapidly metabolized to the nonpsychoactive

11-nor-9-carboxy-THC (THC-COOH). A majority of THC is excreted via the feces (65 percent) with approximately 30 percent of the THC eliminated in the urine as conjugated glucuronic acids and free THC hydroxylated metabolites. At this point, THC becomes inactive or nonpsychoactive.

Pharmacodynamics

The biological effects of cannabinoid compounds, including marijuana, are determined by their binding to and further activation of cannabinoid receptors.[7] Cannabinoids exert their effects by interaction with specific endogenous cannabinoid receptors—CB1 and CB2. The distribution of CB1 follows the pattern of THC and includes cerebral cortex, limbic areas including hippocampus and amygdala, basal ganglia, cerebellum, thalamus, and brain stem. THC increases the release of dopamine from the nucleus accumbens and prefrontal cortex. This effect, which is common to many drugs, such as heroin, cocaine, amphetamine, and nicotine, may be the basis of its reinforcing properties and its recreational use. It is reversed by naloxone, suggesting an opioid link. THC binds to cannabinoid receptors and interferes with important endogenous cannabinoid neurotransmitter systems. Receptor distribution correlates with brain areas involved in physiological, psychomotor, and cognitive effects. As a result, THC produces alterations in motor behavior, perception, cognition, memory, learning, endocrine function, food intake, and regulation of body temperature.

THC is metabolized via cytochrome P450 2C9, 2C11, and 3A isoenzymes. Potential inhibitors of these isoenzymes could decrease the rate of THC elimination if administered concurrently, while potential inducers could increase the rate of elimination.

Effects of Cannabinoids

The euphoria of inhaling cannabinoids comes within minutes of smoking and reaches a plateau lasting two hours or more, depending on dose. There can be dysphoric reactions, such as severe anxiety and panic reactions. Paranoia and psychosis are also dose-related and more common in anxious subjects, "naïve" users, and psychologically vulnerable individuals.

Colors seem brighter, music more vivid, and emotions more poignant and "meaningful." Spatial perception is also distorted. Time perception is impaired, and the ability to know the actual passage of time is flawed. Hallucinations may occur with high doses.

Cannabinoids also affect cognition and psychomotor activities. Effects are consistently dose-related even with long-term users. There is slowing of reaction time, motor incoordination, defects in short-term memory, and difficulty in concentration. There is also impairment in the ability to complete complex tasks that require divided attention. Driving and piloting skills are impaired. Furthermore, these effects are additive and compounded with other central nervous system depressants. Withdrawal symptoms include restlessness, insomnia, anxiety, increased aggression, anorexia, muscle tremor, and autonomic effects.

Physiologic effects influence cardiovascular conditions, such as dose-related tachycardia of up to 160 beats/ minutes or more. With chronic use, although tolerance can develop, widespread vasodilation and reddening of conjunctiva and postural hypotension and fainting can still occur. These effects are risker for individuals with a predisposition to cardiac disease.

Respiratory issues include the herbal cannabis preparation that exposes individuals to more carbon monoxide, bronchial irritants, tumor initiators, tumor promoters, and carcinogens than tobacco smoke— five times greater increase in carboxyhemoglobin, three times greater amount of tar inhaled, and one-third more retention in the respiratory tract of tar than smoking a tobacco cigarette.[8] Chronic cannabis smoking is also associated with increased risks for chronic obstructive pulmonary disease.

Drug Interactions

The issue of cannabis and drug interactions is extensive, and two types of drug interactions are pharmacodynamic and pharmacokinetic.

Pharmacodynamic drug interactions occur when two drugs exhibit similar effects on the body. In this case, the central nervous system (CNS) sedation is the main action of cannabis, and there are a multitude of drugs that can cause CNS sedation: benzodiazepine, antipsychotics, opiates, barbiturates, and others.

Pharmacokinetic drug interactions deal with how one drug can affect the absorption, distribution, metabolism, and/or excretion of another drug. Each drug has a process of how the body "normally" handles the drug's absorption, metabolism, excretion, etc. A drug is absorbed at a specific rate and extent, distributed throughout the body at a certain volume, and metabolized and excreted at a certain rate. In the case of cannabis, it is an inhibitor of one of the main metabolic pathways (CYP3A4), as well as an inducer of another common metabolic pathway (CYP1A2).

If the metabolic pathway is inhibited, the other drugs that use the pathway will not get metabolized at a normal rate, and this can cause potential toxicity of that particular drug. As an example, if a patient takes the anticoagulant warfarin (Coumadin) and decides to smoke marijuana, the warfarin metabolism may be inhibited, and the patient will accumulate a higher concentration of warfarin in the system and will be at risk for excessive bleeding.

If the metabolic pathway is induced, the other drugs that use the pathway will get metabolized at a faster rate that can cause therapeutic failure of the drug.

For example, if a patient takes alprazolam (Xanax) then starts to smoke cannabis, this will lead to a lower concentration of alprazolam, which could to lead to withdrawal and possibly seizures.

Sometimes there could be two different mechanisms at work. In the case of the abovementioned patient, for the first few days, the pharmacodynamic interaction of the additive sedation will predominate, and the patient will be oversedated, but invariably the pharmacokinetic interaction will predominate, resulting in lower serum concentration and less sedation.

Cannabis inhibits the CYP3A4 pathway, so all drugs that use CYP3A4 as a moderate to major pathway could be affected significantly. Furthermore, because a drug inhibits or induces the system does not mean it uses the system, but substrates of CYP3A4 need to be considered. There are many "minor" substrates of this system, but these interactions are not clinically relevant. Also, the likelihood for drugs that are topicals or ophthalmics to interact is very low.

The cannabidiol-rich cannabis extract, CBD, has been shown to be widely effective for children with epilepsy. CBD and conventional anticonvulsant drugs have some similar action mechanisms. CBD has antiseizure effects and better seizure control.[9] It is suggested that CBD may block seizures by blocking the N-methyl-D-aspartate (NMDA) receptor, enhancing the gamma-aminobutyric acid (GABA) receptor, and stabilizing ion channels similar to mechanisms as Banzel, Lamictal, Dilantin, Keppra, and Trileptal.[10] CBD also received orphan drug status in the United States as an orally administered liquid for the treatment of Dravet syndrome.[11] Further research will help determine which types of epilepsy CBD is going to help, its side effects, and how it interacts with other antiseizure drugs.

Summary

Chronic cannabis use results in tolerance, dependence, withdrawal, and long-term cognitive impairments. Long-term use carries respiratory, cardiovascular, and other health risks. Cannabis use is associated with adverse psychosocial problems and affects multiple organ systems. Many physicians, medical organizations, health care providers, government/ elected officials, and individuals take differing views of the benefits and risks of medical cannabis; but almost everyone agrees further research is needed.

Notes

1. Leggett, T. United Nations Office on Drugs and Crime: A review of the world cannabis situation. *Bull Narc.* 2006;58:1.

2. Ashton, C. H. Pharmacology and effects of cannabis: A brief review. *British Journal of Psychiatry.* 2001;178:101–106.

3. Borgelt, L. M., Franson, K. L., Nussbaum, A. M., and Wang, G. S. The pharmacologic and clinical effects of medical cannabis. *Pharmacotherapy* (Review). February 2013;33(2):195–209.

4. Ashton, C. H. Pharmacology and effects of cannabis: A brief review. *British Journal of Psychiatry.* 2001;178:101–106.

5. Bailey, J. A., DuPont, R. L., and Teitelbaum, S. A. Cannabis use disorder: Epidemiology, comorbidity, and pathogenesis. *UpToDate.* August 2013.

6. Ashton, C. H. Pharmacology and effects of cannabis: A brief review. *British Journal of Psychiatry.* 2001;178:101–106.

7. Manzanares, J., Julian, M. D., and Carrascosa, A. Role of the cannabinoid system in pain control and therapeutic implications for the management of acute and chronic pain episodes. *Current Neuropharmacology.* July 2006;4(3):239–257.

8. Ashton, C. H. Pharmacology and effects of cannabis: A brief review. *British Journal of Psychiatry.* 2001;178:101–106.

9. Hill, T. D., et al. Cannabidivarin-rich cannabis extracts are anticonvulsant in mouse and rat via a CB1

receptor-independent mechanism. *British Journal of Pharmacology.* October 2013.

10.   O'Shaughnessy's News Service. Dr. Goldstein on caring for kids with epilepsy. February 2014.

11.   Wilner, A. N. Marijuana for epilepsy: Weighing the evidence. *Medscape Neurology.* WebMD. March 2014.

The Endocannabinoid System in Health and Disease

Thomas Penders, MD, MS, DLFAPA

Introduction

Following the identification and isolation of Δ-9-Tetrahydocannabinnol (THC) as the molecule responsible for the psychoactive effect of marijuana, THC was synthesized and became available to medical researchers in 1964. Prior to these discoveries, it had been known that the cannabis plant contained a variety of chemical products.[1] Today, despite the discovery of 70 such products, THC remains the only one capable of causing mood- or sensory-altering effects. Consequently, medical research has only recently begun to look at the effects of the remaining nonpsychoactive constituents of the cannabis plant.

While exploring the mechanism by which THC exerts its effects on the brain, researchers discovered a naturally occurring system, including lipid-based constituents, capable of producing actions similar to THC. This system of naturally occurring substances is part of what has become known as the endocannabinoid system. This system is present widely throughout the brain and has its own enzyme system regulating production and breakdown of the endogenous components anandamide and 2-arachidonoyol glycerol (2-AG), the primary neurotransmitters for this system. Since 1988, it has been known that these chemical messengers act on specific receptors in the brain that have come to be known as CB receptors.

Cannabinoid Receptor Systems

Currently there is acceptance of two different CB receptors, CB1 and CB2. CB1 receptors are stimulated by the naturally occurring molecules, anandamide and 2-AG. These receptors, by a coincidence of nature, are also partially stimulated by THC. CB1 receptors are located in areas of the brain that serve to coordinate movement (basal ganglia and cerebellum) and are densely present in the area of the brain where memories for emotional events appear to be stored (hippocampus) and where fearful responses are coordinated (amygdala). These receptors are also distributed in areas that serve sensory functions, such as hearing, taste, smell, and touch, and "association areas" where simple sensory functions are coordinated with other brain inputs (frontal cortex). This system of chemical messengers and receptors is unique in that there are no nerve cells or nerve circuits that are regulated purely by the endocannabinoid system. Rather, CB1 receptors exist on nerve cells whose signaling systems are controlled by the more well-known neurotransmitters (i.e., dopamine, serotonin GABA, and acetylcholine). Further, the CB1 receptors exist only on the "presynaptic" part of the nerve cell, the part of the circuit that sends out the chemical signal. More traditional neurotransmitters have their receptors primarily on the "postsynaptic" portion of the nerve terminal, the part of the nerve cell that conveys messages further down the line. It has become clear to those studying this system that the endocannabinoid system exists to help regulate the activity of other neurotransmitter systems. Most commonly, a stimulation of the CB1 receptor will reduce activity and decrease the amount of traditional neurotransmitter released by a nerve cell for a given stimulation. Evidence is increasing then that the endocannabinoid system serves as a kind of break on nerve activity. The system has therefore been characterized as an "antistress" system and may have evolved to protect the nervous system during times of overstimulation or stress. Stimulation of brain CB1 receptors results in many of the perceptual changes that are associated with the psychotropic effects of marijuana.[2]

The CB2 receptors are located largely outside of the brain and have important, though similar, roles in regulating activities of other systems, such as the immune and metabolic system. CB2 receptors exist in large numbers in the spleen, in the bone marrow, in the gastrointestinal system, and on peripheral nerves. The chemical messengers anandamide and 2-AG stimulate the CB2 receptors. Stimulation also tends to inhibit the activity of the cells where these receptors exist. Stimulation of the CB2 receptors produces effects throughout the body that we associate with use of marijuana.[3]

Drugs That Affect the Endocannabinoid System

Over the past quarter century, researchers have been able to synthesize chemical products that have specific actions on the CB1 and CB2 receptors. While the "synthetic cannabinoids" were used originally to help explore the nature of the endocannabinoid system, more recently they have been considered candidates as therapeutic agents that have actions through the natural protective function that seems to be a consistent result of increased activity of the endocannabinoid system. Several years ago, a drug company (Sanofi-Aventis) marketed a drug in Europe that had the effect of reducing appetite. Since stimulation of the CB1 receptor increases appetite (as with the "munchies"), blockade of stimulation of the CB1 receptor decreases appetite. This drug, rimonabant, was indeed an effective agent for weight loss. It also blocked the psychoactive effects of marijuana.[4] The drug, however, was removed from the market after reports of associated anxiety and depression and several suicides relating to use of the drug. Further research is currently being directed at learning more about the role of these receptors in several important psychiatric disorders, such as depression, anxiety, psychoses, and addictions. There is accumulating evidence that hypoaction of the brain endocannabinoid system is associated with depression and that enhanced signaling within the system has antidepressant effects in normal individuals as well as those with depressive illness. More recently, selective activation of CB2 receptors has been shown to reduce the stimulant effects of cocaine.

Synthetic Cannabinoids as Drugs of Abuse

Tragically, many of the chemicals developed by researchers to study the endocannabinoid system have been hijacked by chemists in overseas laboratories and have been manufactured, distributed, and promoted as "synthetic marijuana." These products, commonly referred to as "spice products" or K-2, are today commonly used by youth interested in drug experimentation. The use of these substances that produce much more potent stimulation than THC has resulted in psychotic reactions that may require hospitalization. There is good evidence that use of these drugs by patients with chronic psychotic disorders can produce acute exacerbations in previously stable patients.[5]

Other Constituents of the Cannabis Plant

A different constituent of the cannabis plant, cannabidiol, has been the subject of recent studies. This constituent appears to have effects on the endocannabinoid system that are neuro-protective in nature. This substance may have antiepileptic effects in some. The presence of higher concentrations of cannabidiol in some varieties of the cannabis plant appears to reduce the psychomimetic effect associated with THC. Several workers have suggested that cannabidiol may have potential as an antipsychotic.[6]

Summary

The active agent of marijuana, THC, appears to act on receptors present through the brain and distributed widely throughout the body that are part of a natural system that appears to exist to prevent damage from overstimulation or stress. Increasing knowledge of the mechanisms by which this system operates offers insights into how alterations in function of this system may play a role in psychiatric and medical disorders. Use of drugs that affect the endocannabinoid system will likely become important therapeutic tools in treatment of psychiatric and other disorders in the future.

Notes

1. Gaoni, Y., and Mechoulam, R. Isolation, structure, and synthesis of an active constituent of hashish. *Journal of the American Chemical Society.* 1964;86:1646–1647.

2. Haring, M., Guggenhuber, S., and Lutz, B. Neuronal populations mediating the effects of endocannabinoids on stress and emotionality. *Neuroscience.* 2012;204:145–158.

3. Mechoulam, R., and Parker, L. A. The endocannabinoid system and the brain. *Annual Review of Physiology.* 2013;64:21–47.

4. Vemuri, V. K., Janero, D. R., and Makriyannusis, A. Pharmacotherapeutic targeting of the endocannabinoid signaling system: Drugs for obesity and the metabolic syndrome. *Physiology of Behavior.* 2008;93:671–686.

5. EMCDDA. *Understanding the "spice" phenomenon. Thematic papers.* European Monitoring Centre for Drugs and Drug Addiction. 2009.

6. Isegoer, T. A., and Bossong, M. G. A systematic review of the antipsychotic properties of cannabidiol in humans. *Schizophrenia Research.* 2015;160(1–3):153–161.

Medical Marijuana—Evidence, Accepted Indications, and Current Use

Chelsea L. Neumann, MD, and
Ashwin A. Patkar, MD, DFAPA, MRCPsych

Introduction

The use of marijuana (cannabis) for medical indications remains controversial because of limitations in scientific evidence, state and federal restrictions, and legal status of marijuana. As of November 15, 2014, 23 states and the District of Columbia have legalized marijuana for medical purposes despite US Drug Enforcement Agency (DEA) classification of cannabis as a schedule I drug with no currently accepted medical use and high potential for abuse. Four states and the District have legalized recreational marijuana. Physicians are caught between growing medical research indicating medical potential for $\Delta(9)$-tetrahydrocannabinol (THC) and cannabidiol (CBD) and federal regulations limiting legal prescribing.

In North Carolina, House Bill 1161, introduced on May 20, 2014, if passed would have placed on the November 4, 2014, statewide election ballot, a constitutional amendment to allow the medical use of cannabis. The bill died when the legislature adjourned May 22, 2014, rendering medical marijuana currently illegal in North Carolina. However, a bill was signed and approved by the governor in June 2014 legalizing the use of CBD oil, an extract from the popular strain of cannabis known as Charlotte's Web for intractable epilepsy in North Carolina.

Position Statements of National Medical Associations

The American Medical Association (AMA) stated in June 2001, "The AMA calls for further adequate and well-controlled studies of marijuana and related cannabinoids in patients who have serious conditions for which preclinical, anecdotal, or controlled evidence suggests possible efficacy and the application of such results to the understanding and treatment of disease." In November 2013, the AMA reaffirmed its opposition to marijuana legalization but also called the current federal approach to reducing the drug's use "ineffective" and endorsed a review of the "risks and benefits" of new legal markets in Colorado and Washington. The 2011 position statement by the American Society of Addiction Medicine (ASAM) asserts that "cannabis, cannabis-based products and cannabis delivery devices should be subject to the same standards that are applicable to other prescription medications and medical devices, and that these products should not be distributed to patients unless such products or devices have received marketing approval from the Food and Drug Administration (FDA). ASAM rejects smoking as a means of drug delivery since it is not safe." In 2013, the American Psychiatric Association announced its position statement on marijuana clarifying that "there is no current scientific evidence that marijuana is in any way beneficial for the treatment of any psychiatric disorder. In contrast, current evidence supports, at minimum, a strong association of cannabis use with the onset of psychiatric disorders. Further research on the use of cannabis-derived substances as medicine should be encouraged and facilitated by the federal government. If scientific evidence supports the use of cannabis derived substances to treat specific conditions, the medication should be subject to the approval process of the FDA." A 2004 FDA testimony before the US House of Representatives stated, "Simply having access, without having safety, efficacy, and adequate use information does not help patients," and "FDA will continue to be receptive to sound, scientifically based research into the medicinal uses of botanical marijuana and other cannabinoids."

Synthetic Cannabinoids and Medical Uses

Preparations of the marijuana plant *Cannabis sativa* has been used for centuries in the treatment of rheumatism, convulsions, pain, and other medical indications throughout the world. Of the approximately 60 phytocannabinoids found in cannabis, the two most medically relevant are THC and cannabidiol (CBD), a cannabinoid extract of botanical cannabis. CBD has been shown to have anticonvulsive, sedative, hypnotic, antipsychotic, antinausea, and anti-inflammatory effects.[1]

Chemotherapy-induced nausea and vomiting and AIDS-related wasting syndromes

Synthetic cannabinoids approved by the FDA since 1985 include the cannabinoid (CB1) receptor agonists dronabinol (Marinol) and nabilone (Cesamet). Dronabinol, a schedule III controlled substance, is indicated for chemotherapy-induced nausea and vomiting and AIDS-related anorexia and wasting, with therapeutic effects lasting up to six hours and onset of action 30 to 60 minutes. Nabilone has therapeutic effects that last up to 12 hours, and onset is 60 to 90 minutes. Though synthetic, both THC analogs cause unwanted side effects similar to botanical cannabis, which is associated with euphoria, dysphoria, cognitive slowing, and paranoia. Also, the long onset of action and oral preparation is argued to be less favorable to patients as opposed to immediate onset with inhaled marijuana. A placebo-controlled randomized clinical trial found that in HIV-positive marijuana smokers, both dronabinol (at doses eight times current recommendations) and marijuana (3.9 percent THC) were well tolerated and produced substantial and comparable increases in food intake.[2]

Pain syndromes

Several molecular, biochemical, and pharmacological studies support the existence of reciprocal interactions between the opioid and endocannabinoid systems, suggesting a common underlying mechanism.[3] Furthermore, these systems are thought to work synergistically to enhance analgesia. Recent reviews have indicated a likely future indication for the use of cannabinoids and opioids in tandem for pain and palliative care as a mode of minimizing adverse effects and tolerance associated with the use of opioids alone for analgesia; however, no formal controlled trials support this indication at this time.[4]

The US FDA has expedited a review of Sativex, a medical marijuana spray for the treatment of pain in patients with advanced cancer that is currently in phase 3 trials. Sativex, generic name nabiximols, is composed of CBD and THC in a mucosal spray that is approved in Canada, Mexico, and Europe for the treatment of muscle spasticity caused by multiple sclerosis. Canada also allows the use of Sativex for relief of neuropathic and advanced cancer pain.

Medical marijuana is being used to treat pain associated with a multitude of medical conditions. A recent open-label study found that THC/CBD spray was effective for peripheral neuropathic pain associated with diabetes and allodynia, with half of the patients experiencing at least 30 percent improvement in pain, in addition to improvement in sleep quality.[5] A controlled trial found smoked marijuana was well tolerated and effectively relieved chronic neuropathic pain associated with HIV, concluding its effects were as effective as conventional pain medications.[6] The safety evidence for medical marijuana as a treatment for HIV-associated neuropathic pain and weight loss is mixed, mainly because of concerns that inhaled marijuana may decrease immunity and contribute to opportunistic infections. There is limited evidence for cannabis as treatment for migraines.[7]

Glaucoma

Cannabinoids in smoked marijuana have been shown to reduce intraocular pressure in humans and suggested a therapeutic role in glaucoma.[8] One limitation of smoked marijuana is that it reduces intraocular pressure for only three to four hours, necessitating smoking six to eight times a day and increasing risk of adverse effects. Based on available scientific evidence, the American Academy of Ophthalmology Complementary Therapy Task Force found no scientific evidence demonstrating increased benefit and/or diminished risk of marijuana use in the treatment of glaucoma compared with the wide variety of pharmaceutical agents available.[9] The National Institute on Drug Abuse approved the use of botanical cannabis for glaucoma in 1976, which led to a group of patients receiving treatment until 1992 when the FDA's Compassionate Investigational New Drug Study (CIND) program was suspended.[10] The CIND currently supports the treatment of approximately four patients with federally grown medical cannabis for diagnoses, including glaucoma, multiple sclerosis, nail-patella syndrome, and a rare bone disorder.

Neurological disorders

Evidence supporting the use of medical cannabis for other neurological disorders is mixed. A recent systematic review concluded that oral cannabis extract, THC, and nabiximols were possibly effective for multiple sclerosis–related spasticity and central pain as well as spasms. Nabiximols was probably effective for bladder spasms, though THC and oral cannabis extract was probably not effective. THC and oral cannabis extract was probably ineffective, and nabiximols was possibly ineffective for tremor, and oral cannabinoid extract was probably ineffective for levodopa-induced dyskinesias in Parkinson's disease. The review also concluded oral cannabinoids are of unknown efficacy in non-chorea-related symptoms of Huntington disease, Tourette syndrome, cervical dystonia, and epilepsy and warned of the serious adverse psychological effects of the use of these medications.[11]

A high-concentration CBD:THC strain of cannabis, popularly known as Charlotte's Web, is currently approved for refractory cases of epilepsy in 11 states. This strain gained prominence because of the case study of Charlotte, a five-year-old girl in Colorado with Dravet syndrome, a debilitating gene mutation that contributes to a form of epilepsy that caused her to have over 50 grand mal seizures daily, refractory to conventional antiepileptic medications. After administering CBD oil in a dose of 4 mg CBD/ pound per day, Charlotte's seizures decreased to three seizures per month.[12] Its popularity and touted efficacy has thousands of patients on waiting lists to obtain the oil, traveling across Colorado state lines to obtain the medicine because of its limited availability and high demand. Although there are no available randomized controlled trials of botanical cannabis in epilepsy, anecdotal and survey evidence suggests that it may benefit patients with epilepsy.[13]

Epidiolex is a highly purified CBD containing medication containing no THC extracted from botanical cannabis. Epidiolex has been granted Orphan Drug Designation by the FDA in the treatment of Dravet and Lennox-Gastaut syndromes since November 2013, each of which is a severe childhood-onset drug-resistant epilepsy syndrome. It is manufactured by the UK's GW Pharmaceuticals and is composed of highly purified CBD containing no THC extracted from botanical cannabis. As of October 30, 2014, a worldwide phase 2/3 clinical trial is under way testing the safety and efficacy of Epidiolex in children and adolescents with Dravet syndrome. Epidiolex is considered a schedule I substance by the FDA and is closely monitored and restricted by both the FDA and US Drug Enforcement Agency.[14,15]

Psychiatric disorders

There is strong evidence to suggest that frequent cannabis use is an independent risk factor for emergence of psychosis, and those with established vulnerability are particularly sensitive to its effects, leading to poor outcome.[16,17] A causal relationship between cannabis and schizophrenia has not been firmly established. Given the association between cannabis use and psychosis, individuals at risk for or suffering from schizophrenia or bipolar disorder should be discouraged from marijuana use.[18] However, GW Pharmaceuticals is currently enrolling patients in the UK and Poland in a phase 2a trial to investigate possible antipsychotic properties of a high-potency CBD and low-potency THC compound GWP42003 in patients with schizophrenia, noting on their Web site, "GWP42003 has shown notable anti psychotic effects in accepted pre clinical models of schizophrenia and importantly has also demonstrated the ability to reduce the characteristic movement disorders induced by currently available anti psychotic agents."[19]

Limited evidence from small studies suggests THC may reduce tics and behavioral problems in patients with Tourette syndrome.[20] There is minimal evidence to support use of medical marijuana for symptoms of major depressive disorder, bipolar affective disorder, anxiety disorders, and posttraumatic stress disorder (PTSD), with some evidence suggesting adverse effects of cannabis on these conditions in adolescents.[21,22,23,24]

While biochemically it is believed that the endocannabinoid system, specifically anandamide, may have implications in the extinction of fear, experts are hesitant to claim botanical cannabinoids in their current medicinal form may be useful as treatment for PTSD.[25] Current research indicates only temporary relief may be obtained for individuals with PTSD using currently available cannabinoids as treatment.[26]

There is insufficient evidence indicating positive effects of medical cannabis on symptoms of depression. However, studies indicate significant daily use of marijuana is likely to contribute or exacerbate symptoms of depression.[27] Prospective and retrospective studies have found that marijuana use did not correlate with increased or decreased suicide.[28,29]

Some pilot data show that nabilone may reduce symptoms of marijuana withdrawal. However, current evidence to support use of medical marijuana in marijuana, opioid, or other substance dependence remains insufficient.[30]

Conclusions and Future Directions

Medicinal use of marijuana may benefit selected cases of refractory chemotherapy-induced nausea and vomiting and AIDS-related wasting syndromes and intractable seizures. There is emerging evidence that medical marijuana may also have a role in specific pain syndromes and neurological disorders. However, in all these conditions, there is a clear need for more efficacy and safety research. Pharmacological studies investigating synthetic cannabinoid compounds that can selectively modulate the endocannabinoid system in humans have increased substantially. This may permit better understanding of the effects of THC and CBD on the individual CB1 and CB2 receptors and can clarify the potential medicinal effects of these chemicals.

The health risks posed by smoking marijuana, the challenges of dose administration by smoking, and the negative psychological effects associated with ingesting and smoking botanical cannabis limit acceptability and safe prescribing by the medical profession. Clinical research in medicinal use of marijuana can improve our understanding of potential positive effects as well as the risk and safety of the product. Such research can help clinicians, patients, policy makers, and the public to make informed decisions regarding the role of medical marijuana.

Notes

1. Luvone, et al. Neuroprotective effect of cannabidiol, a non-psychoactive component from *Cannabis sativa*,

on B-amyloid-induced toxicity in PC12 cells. *Journal of Neurochemistry.* 2004.

2. Haney, et al. Dronabinol and marijuana in HIV-positive marijuana smokers: Caloric intake, mood, and sleep. *Journal of Acquired Immune Deficiency Syndromes.* August 15, 2007.

3. Desroches, et al. Opioids and cannabinoids interactions: Involvement in pain management. *Curr Drug Targets.* April 2010;11(4):462–73.

4. McCarberg, B. H. Cannabinoids: Their role in pain and palliation. *J Pain Palliat Care Pharmacother.* 2007;21(3):19–28.

5. Hoggart, et al. A multicentre, open-label, follow-on study to assess the long-term maintenance of effect, tolerance, and safety of THC/CBD oromucosal spray in the management of neuropathic pain. *J Neurol.* September 30, 2014.

6. Abrams, et al. Smoked cannabis therapy for HIV-related painful peripheral neuropathy: Results of a randomized,

placebo-controlled clinical trial. September 9–10, 2005. Abstract presented at the International Association for Cannabis as Medicine 3rd Conference on Cannabinoids in Medicine.

7. McGeeney, B. E. Cannabinoids and hallucinogens for headache. *Headache.* March 2013;53(3):447–58.

8. Tomida, et al. Cannabinoids and glaucoma. *Br J Ophthalmol.* May 2004;88(5):708–13. Review.

9. American Academy of Ophthalmology. Complementary therapy assessment: Marijuana in the treatment of glaucoma. June 2014.

10. Seamon, M. J. The legal status of medical marijuana. *Ann Pharmacother.* 2006;40(12):2211–2215.

11. Koppel, et al. Systematic review: Efficacy and safety of medical marijuana in selected neurologic disorders. Report of the Guideline Development Subcommittee of the American Academy of Neurology. *Neurology.* April 29, 2014;82(17):1556–63.

12. Maa, et al. The case for medical marijuana in epilepsy. *Epilepsia.* June 2014;55(6):783–6.

13. Gross, et al. Marijuana use and epilepsy: Prevalence in patients of a tertiary care epilepsy center. *Neurology.* June 8, 2014.

14. http://www.gwpharm.com/Epidiolex.aspx

15. http://clinicaltrials.gov/ct2/show/ NCT02224703?term=epidiolex+dravet&rank=1

16. Bostwick, J. M. Blurred boundaries: The therapeutics and politics of medical marijuana. 2012 Mayo Foundation for Medical Education and Research. *Mayo Clin Proc.* 2012;87(2):172–186.

17. Foti, et al. Cannabis use and the course of schizophrenia: 10-year follow-up after first hospitalization. *Am J Psychiatry.* August 2010;167(8):987–993.

18. Henquet, et al. Psychosis reactivity to cannabis use in daily life: An experience sampling study. *Br J Psychiatry.* June 2010; 196(6):447–453.

19. http://www.gwpharm.com/psychiatric-conditions. aspx

20. Müller-Vahl, K. R. Treatment of Tourette syndrome with cannabinoids. *Behav Neurol.* 2013;27(1):119–24.

21. Degenhardt, et al. The persistence of the association between adolescent cannabis use and common mental disorders into young adulthood. *Addiction.* January 2013;108(1):124–33.

22. Duffy, et al. Adolescent substance use disorder during the early stages of bipolar disorder: A prospective high-risk study. *J Affect Disord.* December 15, 2012;142(1–3):57–64.

23. Lynskey, et al. Major depressive disorder, suicidal ideation, and suicide attempt in twins discordant for cannabis dependence and early-onset cannabis use. *Arch Gen Psychiatry.* October 2004;61(10):1026–32.

24. Office of National Drug Control Policy, Executive Office of the President. Teen marijuana use worsens depression: An analysis of recent data shows

"self-medicating" could actually make things worse. 2008.

25. Chhatwal, et al. Enhancing cannabinoid neurotransmission augments the extinction of conditioned fear. *Neuropsychopharmacology.* March 2005;30(3):516–24.

26. Bowers, et al. Interaction between the cholecystokinin and endogenous cannabinoid systems in cued fear expression and extinction retention. *Neuropsychopharmacology.* September 1, 2014.

27. Lev-ran, et al. The association between cannabis use and depression: A systematic review and meta-analysis of longitudinal studies. *Psychol Med.* March 2014;44(4):797–810.

28. Price, et al. Cannabis and suicide: Longitudinal study. *Br J Psychiatry.* December 2009;195(6):492–7.

29. Rylander, et al. Does the legalization of medical marijuana increase completed suicide? *Am J Drug Alcohol Abuse.* July 2014;40(4):269–73.

30.   Haney, et al. <u>Nabilone decreases marijuana withdrawal and a laboratory measure of marijuana relapse.</u> *Neuropsychopharmacology.* July 2013;38(8):1557–65.

Dr. Neumann and Dr. Patkar have no financial conflicts related to this article.

Correspondence:

Ashwin A. Patkar, MD, MRCPsych

Professor of Psychiatry and Community and Family Medicine

Medical Director, Duke Addictions Programs and Duke Center for Addictive Behavior and Change

2218 Elder St, suite 127

Durham, NC 27705

Tel: 919-668-3626

Fax: 919-668-5418

E-mail: ashwin.patkar@duke.edu

The Social Costs of Marijuana, the Most Frequently Used Illegal Drug in the World

Heather N. Oxentine, MD

The possession, sale, or use of marijuana or products of the *Cannabis sativa* plant had been, until recently, a violation of federal and state laws. The World Health Organization estimates that about 147 million people or 2.5 percent of the world population consume cannabis annually.[1] In 2012, it was estimated that about 12.1 percent of the population over age 12 in the United States had used marijuana within the prior year. Estimated street prices for marijuana in the United States are estimated to range from $10 to $12 per gram as of 2013.[2]

Marijuana-Related Incarceration

In 2012, 42 percent of drug arrests in the United States were for possession of marijuana, and 5.9 percent were for the sale or production of marijuana.[3] Specifically, 749,825 individuals were arrested in the United States for a marijuana law violation, and of those, 658,231 (roughly 88 percent) were arrested for possession solely.[4] In North Carolina law, enforcement made 20,983 marijuana arrests in 2010 (the 10th most in the nation), and marijuana possession arrests accounted for 53.6 percent of all drug arrests in North Carolina during that year.[5] Sixty-two percent of marijuana possession arrests in 2010 were of individuals 24 years old or younger, and more than 34 percent were teenagers or younger.[6] Of interest, the United States accounts for 5 percent of the world's population and accounts for 25 percent of the world's prison population.[7]

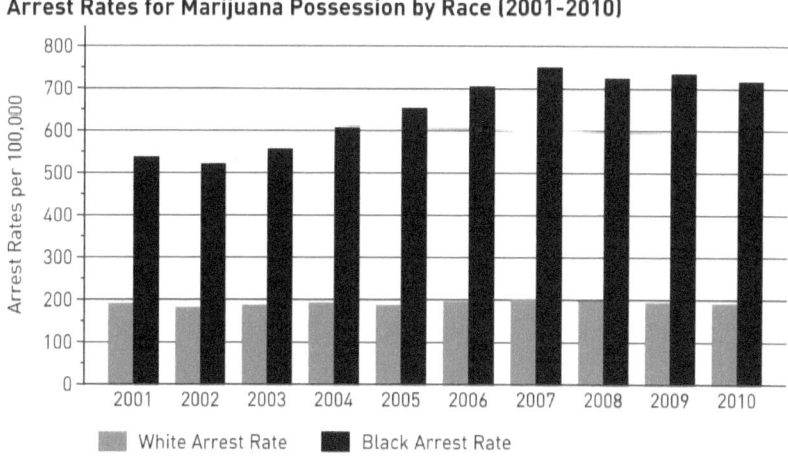

Arrest Rates for Marijuana Possession by Race (2001-2010)

Source: FBI/Uniform Crime Reporting Program Data and U.S. Census Data

Costs to Law Enforcement and Taxpayers

It has been estimated that the total national cost of enforcing marijuana possession laws is approximately $3.613 billion annually. In 2010, it was estimated that states spent $1.747 billion policing marijuana possession arrests, $1.371 billion adjudicating marijuana possession cases, and $495 million incarcerating individuals for marijuana possession.[8] The documentation of racial differentials in the arrests and prosecution of marijuana-related violations has been a source of considerable controversy.

The State of North Carolina spent roughly $55 million enforcing marijuana possession laws in 2010.[9] Many jurisdictions have begun to soften the penalties for possession of small quantities of cannabis and focus on imprisonment for those who traffic the drug on the black market. With the amounts being spent annually on enforcing marijuana laws, some proponents for legalization suggest these amounts could potentially be saved annually if marijuana use was legalized and taxed like tobacco. An analysis from 2005 performed by Jeffrey Miron estimated that if the United States were to legalize marijuana, it would save $7.7 billion in law enforcement costs and generate as much as $6.2 billion annually if marijuana were taxed. A US study from 2006 demonstrated that cannabis was the no. 4 value crop, and even no. 1 or 2 in many states, including California, New York, and Florida, averaging $3,000/lb., placing production at a value of $35.8 billion.[10]

Recent Legalization

In 2012, Washington and Colorado became the first states to officially legalize cannabis under state law.[11] At a federal level, marijuana is still considered illegal and is classified still as a schedule I substance under the Controlled Substances Act, which classifies these substances as having high potential for dependency and no accepted medical use. In August 2013, the US Department of Justice issued a revised memorandum to federal prosecutors, making it clear that marijuana is still an illegal drug under the Controlled Substances Act and will continue to be strictly enforced, specifically naming eight priority enforcement areas. It also addresses the need for state and local authorities to continue to enforce the regulatory efforts at their end.[12] Distribution and use of marijuana remain today a violation of federal law. This includes use of medical marijuana or the use of cannabis and its constituent cannabinoids, such as tetrahydrocannabinol (THC) and cannabidiol (CBD), for medical therapy.

In 1996, California passed Proposition 215, which made the state the first in the union to allow for the medical usage of marijuana. Currently, 23 states, the District of Columbia, and Guam have passed medical marijuana laws.[13]

In 2014, North Carolina passed House Bill 1220 (Epilepsy Alternative Treatment Act), which allows for use of product with low THC/high CBD (cannabidiol oil) in those with intractable epilepsy. The bill authorizes neurologists registered with the Intractable Epilepsy Alternative Treatment Pilot Study to dispense hemp extract acquired outside North Carolina to treat children with intractable epilepsy. The main purpose of the bill was to allow families who have traveled to Colorado to obtain the hemp extract to return back to North Carolina and legally continue the treatment. The bill also encourages the University of North Carolina at Chapel Hill, Duke University, Wake Forest University, and East Carolina University to research hemp oil.[14]

Research on the drug has been difficult to conduct since the plant is illegal in most countries. The cannabis that is available for research studies in the United States is grown at the University of Southern Mississippi and controlled by the National Institute for Drug Abuse.[15] With the recent legalization of medical marijuana in numerous states, many questions are being raised, including how to regulate its recommendation, dispensing, and registration of approved patients.

New concerns with legalization include "drugged driving," which is considered operating a motor vehicle while under the influence of marijuana or other drugs, which can lead to drivers being charged with DUIs similarly as one would with alcohol. In Colorado, impaired driving is considered five nanograms of active THC per milliliter of whole blood. THC has been shown to be associated with poorer driving performance, longer response times, and slower driving speeds. Several studies have actually shown an increase in crash risk in drivers using cannabis. One study found that between 1999 and 2010, the number of drivers testing positive for cannabinol involved in fatal vehicular accidents had tripled.[16] Statistics from 2013 in Colorado show 36 persons testing positive for cannabis alone (5.7 percent) involved in fatal crashes.[17] Prospective monitoring of numbers of accidents, fatalities, and DUIs should provide a measure of the harm associated with liberalization of public policy related to marijuana.

Notes

1. Cannabis. (n.d.). Retrieved January 31, 2015, from http://www.who.int/substance_abuse/facts/cannabis/en/. World Drug Report 2014.

2. (n.d.). Retrieved January 31, 2015, from http://www.unodc.org/documents/wdr2014/Cannabis_2014_web.pdf

3. Crime in the United States 2011. (August 9, 2012). Retrieved January 31, 2015, from http://www.fbi.gov/about-us/cjis/ucr/crime-in-the-u.s/2011/crime-in-the-u.s.-2011/persons-arrested/persons-arrested

4. The War on Marijuana in Black and White. (June 2013). Retrieved January 31, 2015, from https://www.aclu.org/sites/default/files/assets/1114413-mj-report-rfs-rel1.pdf

5. ACLU of North Carolina. (n.d.). Retrieved January 31, 2015, from http://www.acluofnorthcarolina.org/

6. American Civil Liberties Union. (n.d.). Retrieved January 31, 2015, from https://www.aclu.org/

7. Liptak, A. (April 23, 2008). U.S. prison population dwarfs that of other nations. Retrieved January 31, 2015, from http://www.nytimes.com/2008/04/23/world/americas/23iht-23prison.12253738.html?pagewanted=all&_r=0

8. ACLU of North Carolina. (n.d.). Retrieved January 31, 2015, from http://www.acluofnorthcarolina.org/

9. American Civil Liberties Union. (n.d.). Retrieved January 31, 2015, from https://www.aclu.org/

10. Venkataraman, N. (December 18, 2006). Marijuana called top U.S. cash crop. Retrieved January 31, 2015, from http://abcnews.go.com/business/story?id=2735017&page=1

11. Cannabis (drug). (n.d.). Retrieved January 31, 2015, from http://en.wikipedia.org/wiki/Cannabis_(drug)

12. Cole, James M. Memorandum for all United States attorneys. U.S. Department of Justice. Washington, DC. August 29, 2013.

13. American Civil Liberties Union. (n.d.). Retrieved January 31, 2015, from https://www.aclu.org/

14. Canada, K. (June 25, 2014). NewsObserver. com. Retrieved January 31, 2015, from http://www. newsobserver.com/2014/06/25/3964314_house-bill-legalizing-hemp-oil.html?rh=1

15. Cannabis (drug). (n.d.). Retrieved January 31, 2015, from http://en.wikipedia.org/wiki/Cannabis_(drug)

16. Brady, J., and Li, G. Trends in alcohol and other drugs detected in fatally injured drivers in the United States, 1999–2010. *American Journal of Epidemiology.* 2014;180(8):862–863.

17. Safety. (n.d.). Retrieved January 31, 2015, from https:// www.codot.gov/safety/alcohol-and-impaired-driving/ druggeddriving

Neurocognitive Effects of Adolescent Cannabis Use

P.G. Shelton, MD, FAPA

Neurocognitive effects of cannabis use during critical sensitive periods of brain development have been a growing area of research over the last decade. This is likely caused by the increase in cannabis use and the changing public perception of the risks of use of these products. Increased acceptance of cannabis is evidenced by legalization of marijuana for recreation purposes in several states, including Alaska, Colorado, Washington, and Washington, DC. It is also likely that legalization efforts have resulted in an increased perception of safety among cannabis products.

These shifts in public opinion have also led to increasing use of marijuana among the adolescent and young adult population. Cannabis is now the second most used drug after alcohol in this age group with almost 23 percent of high school seniors and 20 percent of college students reporting monthly use in recent surveys.[1] Of even greater concern is the frequency of moderate to heavy use among this population. Such use is increasing with 6.5 percent of high school seniors reporting daily use, compared with just 2.4 percent in 1993.

Adolescence and early adulthood is a time of substantial neurodevelopmental change in the brain, primarily involving pruning mechanisms. The development during this period especially affects the frontal regions involved with executive functioning and higher-order thinking. Consequently, the brain may be more sensitive during these years to externally induced changes in any major neurotransmitter concentrations, such as the endocannabinoid system. This means that research investigating the neurocognitive effects among all levels of use in this age group is an important public health concern. Research in this age group has primarily focused on individuals who started their use as teenagers and those who use regularly, commonly defined as using at least once weekly. Typically, these studies have focused on the changes in individuals' cognitive effects, brain structure, or blood flow and function within the brain.

There is mounting evidence suggesting that regular cannabis use during the teenage or early adult years (between ages 25 and 30) is associated with cognitive deficits. These deficits can affect many different areas within the frontal lobe resulting in observable changes on psychological tests.

One recently published report of a large prospective longitudinal study by Meier and colleagues described the effects on overall IQ scores among more than 1,000 individuals from birth to age 38, including 153 participants with a cannabis use disorder.[2] This study found that among those individuals who used cannabis regularly, there was a 6.6-point change in IQ over those who were not regular users of these products. After controlling for confounding variables, they further discovered explicit deficits in attention span, psychomotor speed, verbal memory, and executive functioning. At least two other eight-year-long longitudinal studies have demonstrated a decline in verbal memory and attention. A strong majority of multiple cross-sectional studies support reductions in processing speed, complex attention, verbal memory, and executive functioning, including risk-taking behavior among frequent marijuana users.[3,4]

Many studies to date have also documented abnormalities in brain structure within both gray and white matters in the brain. These abnormalities may signal neurodevelopmental delays and a disturbance in normal pruning and branching mechanisms, essential to development of the normal adolescent and adult brain. Studies have found increases in the posterior prefrontal cortex, anterior cerebellum, posterior inferior cerebellar vermis, and striatal volumes. Other findings include decreases in the right medial orbitofrontal volumes. Both growth and reduction of hippocampal and amygdala volumes have been seen. These volumetric deviations are likely detrimental as they have been associated with poor executive functioning, poor verbal memory, increased mood symptoms, and novelty-seeking behavior.

Cortical thickness has also been examined among cannabis users by Lopez-Larson and colleagues. They found decreased thickness in the bilateral superior frontal, bilateral insula, and right caudal middle frontal cortices while discovering increased thicknesses in the paracentral, lingual, temporal, and inferior parietal areas comparable with noncannabis users. Finally, Mata and colleagues found reduced cortical gyrification in prefrontal cortex regions in young adult cannabis users compared with nonusing controls.

While cannabinoid receptors are found primarily in the neuronal synapse, they are also present on glial cells that make up the white matter of the brain. Poorer white matter is related to slower processing speed and psychological dysregulation. Such reductions in white matter have been observed in numerous structures within the brains of cannabis users. Bava and colleagues identified seven different white matter tracts affected by regular cannabis use with comorbid alcohol use disorders. These tracts included the bilateral superior longitudinal fasciculus, bilateral thalamic fibers, right superior temporal gyrus, right inferior longitudinal fasciculus, and left posterior corona radiata.

Unfortunately, the alcohol-induced component to these changes could not be quantified. Several more studies, however, have reported reduced white matter quality in several prefrontal cortex, limbic, parietal, and cerebellar tracts in young cannabis users after controlling for use of alcohol. Overall the evidence is in support of significant changes in white and gray matters among regular cannabis users. These changes in brain structure offer concrete evidence that regular cannabis use contributes to anatomical alterations within major structures of the brain.

Cannabis use has also been linked with reductions in cerebral blood flow and inefficient brain activation patterns. Specifically, reductions in cerebral blood flow in the prefrontal cortex, insular, and temporal regions have been observed. It is unknown whether these reductions are partly responsible for the gray and white matter anomalies observed in youth who routinely use cannabis. Additionally, fMRI and PET studies in adolescent cannabis users have found abnormal prefrontal cortex, parietal, insular, limbic, and cerebellar activation during attentional control, finger tapping, spatial and verbal working memory, verbal learning, pleasant stimuli, and executive functioning.

In summary, many studies to date have suggested that regular exposure to exogenous cannabinoids may disrupt normal neurodevelopment. Numerous changes in brain vascularization, activation, gray matter, and white matter are observed. Of all the changes observed, the reduced IQ of nearly half a standard deviation along with decreases in attention span, memory, and executive functioning are perhaps the most significant. Studies point toward some partial recovery in functioning with sustained abstinence in adulthood, but the largest and most significant study to date by Meier and associates showed that younger adolescents never fully returned to their predicted pre-use IQ trajectory.

Currently, researchers are unsure of what levels of routine use and at what age one begins such use in adolescence, if any, would be considered safe from a neurocognitive recovery standpoint. Research and exploration into these questions may be useful goals for future studies. Preventive educational efforts should include the current and compelling evidence that exists showing routine cannabis use, defined as at least once weekly, is not safe and that no level of routine use has been determined to be harmless.

Notes

1. Johnston, L. D., O. P. *Monitoring the future national results on adolescent drug use: Overview of key findings*. Ann Arbor: Institute for Social Research, University of Michigan, 2012.

2. Meier, M. H., C. A. Persistent cannabis users show neuropsychological decline from childhood to midlife. *Proc Natl Acad Sci USA*. 2012;109(40):2657–64.

3. Tapert, S. F., G. E. Substance use and withdrawal: Neuropsychological functioning over 8 years in youth. *J Int Neuropsychol Soc*. 2002;8(7):873–83.

4. Tait, R. J., M. A. Cannabis use and cognitive function: 8-year trajectory in a young adult cohort. *Addiction*. 2011;106(12):2195–203.